ATKINS DIET FOR SENIORS:

Rejuvenate Your Health to
Achieve Optimal Wellness and Longevity

Sarah Rooney

First Edition: **May 2023**

TABLE OF CONTENT

INTRODUCTION..10

Introduction and Overview...............................10

About this Book...11

Who Should Read This Book?........................12

How to Make Use of This Book......................14

Make your meal plan your own:.......................14
Try the recipes: 14
Make a grocery list: 14
Stay motivated:..15
UNDERSTANDING THE ATKINS DIET 16

What exactly is the Atkins Diet? 16

Phase 1: 16
Phase 2: 16
Phase 3: 17
Phase 4: 17
The Atkins Diet in Action 18

The Science Behind the Atkins Diet.............19

Benefits of the Atkins Diet for Seniors 22

Weight loss:..22
Blood sugar control:...23
Cardiovascular health:..23
Brain health: 23
Improved energy and vitality: 23
High blood pressure:..24

Arthritis: 24

Digestive problems: 24

The Atkins Diet's Risks and Limitations for Seniors **25**

Nutrient deficiencies: 25

Kidney function: 26

Dehydration: 26

Adherence issues: 26

MODIFYING THE ATKINS DIET FOR SENIORS **28**

Seniors' Specific Nutritional Needs **28**

Adequate protein: 28

Increased fiber: 28

Sufficient hydration: 28

Adequate vitamin and mineral intake: 28

Limit your salt intake: 29

Calcium: 30

Vitamin D: **30**

Vitamin B12: 30

Potassium: 30

Omega-3 fatty acids: 30

Adapting the Atkins Diet for Seniors **31**

Carbohydrate consumption should be adjusted to: 31

Increasing protein consumption: 31

Incorporating nutrient-dense foods: 32

Keeping hydrated: 32

Collaboration with a healthcare professional: 32

Calculating Your Daily Carbohydrate Intake **33**

Determine your daily calorie requirements: 33

Calculate your carbohydrate intake: 33

Calculate your daily carbohydrate consumption: 33

Track your carbohydrate consumption: 34

Diet tips that make it easier to stick to 36

Meal planning: 36

Cooking in bulk: 36

Experiment with new meals: 37

Drink Water: 37

Seek help: 37

EATING ON THE ATKINS DIET 38

Meal preparation on the Atkins Diet 38

Protein-rich foods: 38

Include low-carb veggies 38

Make a plan: 39

Keep track of your progress: 39

Portion management is essential: 39

Experiment with recipes: 39

Drink Water: 39

Consider supplements: 40

Atkins Recipes for Seniors 40

Breakfast 40

Grilled Salmon with Asparagus and Cauliflower Rice 40

Chicken Broccoli Alfredo 42

Zucchini Noodle Lasagna 43

Grilled Salmon with Asparagus 45

Greek Salad with Grilled Chicken 46

Zucchini Noodles with Meat Sauce 48

Grilled Salmon with Mango Salsa.. 50

Quinoa Salad with Roasted Vegetables 51

Turkey and Vegetable Stir-Fry.. 53

Grilled Salmon with Avocado Salsa 55

Recipes for Lunch.. 57

Quinoa and Vegetable Salad 57

Chickpea and Sweet Potato Stew 58

Tuna Salad with Greek Yogurt....................................... 60

Grilled Chicken and Quinoa Salad:.................................. 61

Tuna Avocado Lettuce Wraps: 62

Chickpea and Veggie Bowl: 64

Grilled Chicken Salad: 65

Quinoa and Black Bean Bowl:... 67

Tuna and Egg Salad:.. 68

Recipes for Dinner.. 70

Grilled Lemon Herb Chicken 70

Baked Salmon with Asparagus... 71

Grilled Salmon with Asparagus.. 73

Baked Chicken with Broccoli and Cheese 74

Beef and Broccoli Stir-Fry 76

Grilled Salmon with Avocado Salsa 77

Spicy Shrimp Stir-Fry 79

Grilled Chicken with Roasted Vegetables 80

Garlic Ginger Baked Salmon.. 82

Grilled Chicken and Vegetables Skewers 84

Stuffed Portobello Mushrooms.. 86

Apple Slices with Almond Butter and Cinnamon.................... 88

Greek Yogurt with Berries and Honey 89

Recipes for Snacks **90**

Greek Yogurt and Berry Parfait: 90

Veggie Sticks with Hummus: 91

Apple Slices with Almond Butter: 92

Apple Nachos 92

Roasted Chickpeas 93

Cucumber Hummus Bites 95

Greek Yogurt Dip: 96

Apple Slices with Almond Butter: 97

Greek Yogurt and Fruit Parfait 98

Apple Slices with Almond Butter and Cinnamon 99

Greek Yogurt with Berries and Honey 100

Shopping List: **101**

Protein: 102

Vegetables: 102

Fruits: 103

Pantry Staples: 103

Dairy: 104

Eggs: 104

Miscellaneous: 105

STAYING ON TRACK **106**

Mindset and Motivation **106**

Create attainable objectives: 106

Maintain a food journal: 107

Make a plan: 107

Maintain contact: 107

Celebrate your accomplishments: 107

Overcoming Obstacles **108**

Maintain a good attitude: 108

Set attainable objectives:..108

Create a strategy: 108

Seek help:..109

Self-care: 109

Stay adaptable: 109

Seek help and accountability:.......................................109

Maintain your flexibility and adaptability: 110

Including Exercise in the Atkins Diet................................. 111

Begin Slowly· 111

Choose Activities You Will Enjoy: 111

Find a Workout Partner:...111

Change It Up: 111

Make it a habit: 112

Fuel your exercises:..112

Habits of a Healthy Lifestyle 115

Regular physical activity: 115

Staying hydrated:..116

Sleep:..116

Stress management: 116

Mindful eating:..116

Balanced meals:..117

Portion control:..117

HEALTH BENEFITS OF THE ATKINS DIET FOR SENIORS........... 118

Weight loss and weight management 118

Set attainable weight reduction goals:...........................118

Keep track of your progress:..118

Make good food choices:...119

Exercise on a daily basis: 119

Drink enough water: 119

Get adequate sleep: 119

Manage stress: 120

Blood Sugar Control **120**

Balanced Meals: 120

Portion Control: 121

Exercise on a regular basis: 121

Stress Management: 121

Adequate Sleep: 121

Heart Health **122**

Adapting the Atkins Diet for Medical Conditions **123**

CONCLUSION **126**

Key Principles and Strategies: Recap **126**

Motivation to Get Started 127

Final Thoughts and Success Strategies **129**

Set attainable objectives: 129

Keep track of your progress: 129

Plan your meals: 129

Find assistance: 130

INTRODUCTION

I want to start by saying thank you for choosing this book. I hope you found it insightful and helpful.

Introduction and Overview

The Atkins Diet for Seniors welcomes you to the wonderful world of better health and fitness! You've come to the perfect spot if you're a senior trying to take charge of your health and manage your weight. We've looked at how the Atkins Diet may provide a personalized and successful approach to low-carbohydrate eating, adapted particularly to the demands and problems of seniors.

You can expect a thorough and practical guide to the Atkins Diet for Seniors, replete with tailored meal plans, tasty and healthy recipes, shopping lists, and recommendations for remaining motivated and on track, thanks to our high-level table of contents.

Whether you want to lose weight, control your blood sugar levels, or lower your risk of chronic conditions like diabetes, heart disease, and hypertension, this book will provide you with the knowledge and skills you need to succeed.

So, come along with us on this path to better health and fitness with the Atkins Diet for Seniors.

About this Book

The Atkins Diet for Elders is a thorough guide to implementing a low-carbohydrate diet that is customized to the specific nutritional demands and obstacles that elders experience. This book provides a scientifically supported and practical method for attaining your health and weight reduction objectives, with an emphasis on personalization, sustainability, and fun.

This book contains in-depth information on the science behind the Atkins Diet, its potential advantages for seniors, and how to tailor the diet to your specific requirements. You'll also find tasty and healthy recipes for every meal of the day, as well as advice on meal planning, grocery shopping, and keeping motivated.

The Atkins Diet for Seniors provides a sustainable and pleasurable approach to low-carbohydrate eating, whether you want to lose weight, regulate your blood sugar levels, or minimize your risk of chronic conditions including diabetes, heart disease, and hypertension. This book is for you if you're ready to take charge of your health and alter your life.

Who Should Read This Book?

The Atkins Diet for Seniors is a thorough handbook written exclusively for seniors who want to enhance their health and manage their weight by following a low-carbohydrate diet. This book is intended for seniors who want to lose weight, regulate their blood sugar levels, or lower their risk of chronic conditions including diabetes, heart disease, and hypertension.

This book is intended especially for seniors who may be suffering from age-related changes in their health, such as a slowed metabolism, decreased muscle mass, or changes in nutritional absorption. These changes might make maintaining a healthy weight and managing chronic health issues difficult for seniors. The Atkins Diet for Elders is a specialized approach to low-carbohydrate eating that is geared particularly to the nutritional demands and obstacles that elders encounter.

This book is also appropriate for seniors who want to understand the science behind the Atkins Diet and how it works to encourage weight reduction, reduce inflammation, and enhance metabolic health. It includes thorough instructions on how to adapt the Atkins Diet to fit the specific needs of seniors, as well as advice on meal planning, grocery shopping, and remaining motivated.

Overall, the Atkins Diet for Seniors is for any senior who wants to take charge of their health and improve their quality of life by eating low-carbohydrate foods in a sustainable and pleasurable way. Whether you're a novice or a seasoned dieter, this book provides practical guidance, delectable recipes, and a complete guide to reaching your health and weight reduction objectives.

How to Make Use of This Book

The Atkins Diet for Seniors is intended to be a realistic and user-friendly program for seniors to follow in order to enhance their health and control their weight. Here are some pointers on how to get the most out of this book:

Make your meal plan your own: The book offers customizable meal plans that you may modify to meet your own requirements and interests. Use these meal plans as a starting point and make changes as needed to suit your objectives.

Try the recipes: The book includes recipes for every meal of the day, as well as snacks and desserts. To keep your meals interesting and entertaining, try these recipes and experiment with your own versions.

Make a grocery list: To make food shopping easier and more effective, use the shopping lists supplied in the book. These lists are intended to assist you in selecting nutritious meals that are low in carbs.

Stay motivated: The book contains tactics and advice for staying motivated and on track with your diet. Use these suggestions to overcome obstacles and remain dedicated to your health and weight reduction objectives.

Overall, the Atkins Diet for Seniors is a thorough program for seniors to follow in order to adopt a low-carbohydrate diet, improve their health, and control their weight. Whether you're a novice or an experienced dieter, this book will help you reach your objectives by providing practical guidance, delicious recipes, and a customized meal plan.

CHAPTER ONE

UNDERSTANDING THE ATKINS DIET

What exactly is the Atkins Diet?

Dr. Robert Atkins invented the Atkins Diet in the 1970s, which is a low-carbohydrate, high-fat diet. The diet is based on the idea that eating less carbohydrate and more fat might help the body burn stored fat for energy, resulting in weight reduction and better metabolic health.

The Atkins Diet is divided into four stages that gradually reintroduce carbs into the diet:

Phase 1: In this phase, carbohydrate intake is limited to 20–25 grams per day, and high-fat meals are prioritized. This phase usually lasts two weeks and is intended to jumpstart weight reduction.

Phase 2: Balancing: During this phase, carbohydrate intake is gradually raised by 5 grams per week with the objective of achieving "carbohydrate equilibrium," the carbohydrate intake amount at which weight reduction is still accomplished.

Phase 3: Fine-tuning: Carbohydrate consumption is raised further, but at a slower rate, with the objective of long-term weight management.

Phase 4: The diet becomes a long-term lifestyle, with the objective of preserving weight loss and excellent health.

The Atkins Diet emphasizes full, unprocessed meals like meat, fish, eggs, and vegetables while restricting or eliminating refined carbs like bread, pasta, and sugary foods. In addition, the diet promotes the use of healthy fats such as olive oil, avocados, and almonds.

Although the Atkins Diet has been proven to be successful for weight reduction and metabolic health, it may not be appropriate for everyone. Before beginning the Atkins Diet, like with any other diet, it is critical to check with a healthcare physician.

The Atkins Diet in Action

The Atkins Diet increases the burning of stored fat for energy by producing a state of ketosis in the body. When carbohydrate consumption is restricted, the body switches to using fat for fuel rather than glucose from carbs.

When carbohydrate consumption is reduced, the body begins to break down stored fat into molecules known as ketones, which are then utilized for energy by the body. This mechanism results in weight reduction because the body burns fat for fuel rather than storing it.

The Atkins Diet also aids in blood sugar stabilization by limiting the consumption of high-glycemic carbs, which can cause blood sugar to rise and fall. People with type 2 diabetes or prediabetes may benefit the most from this.

Another advantage of the Atkins Diet is that it can help to lessen hunger and cravings since high-fat foods are more satiating and can keep you feeling full for longer periods of time.

The Atkins Diet is usually followed in four stages, with each phase progressively reintroducing carbs into the diet. This helps the body respond to variations in macronutrient ratios and can aid in the prevention of negative effects such as tiredness and headaches.

Overall, the Atkins Diet can be a good approach to losing weight and improving metabolic health, but it is not for everyone. Before beginning the Atkins Diet, like with any other diet, it is critical to check with a healthcare physician.

The Science Behind the Atkins Diet

The Atkins Diet's science is founded on the notion of carbohydrate restriction and its impact on the body's metabolism.

Carbohydrates are broken down into glucose and delivered into the circulation when ingested. This causes the pancreas to produce insulin, which aids in the transfer of glucose into cells for energy. When carbs are ingested in excess, the body may develop insulin resistance, resulting in elevated blood sugar levels and an increased risk of developing type 2 diabetes.

The Atkins Diet limits carbohydrate consumption, lowering insulin requirements and encouraging the breakdown of stored fat for energy. Weight loss and better metabolic health indicators, such as insulin sensitivity, blood sugar management, and cholesterol profile, can result from this.

The Atkins Diet has been proven in studies to be helpful for weight reduction and improving metabolic health. A 2018 meta-analysis of 32 randomized controlled studies, for example, showed that low-carbohydrate diets, including the Atkins Diet, were more successful for weight reduction than low-fat diets over a 12-month period.

Furthermore, according to a 2019 study published in the journal Nutrients, a low-carbohydrate diet comparable to the Atkins Diet was successful in improving glycemic control and lowering medication use in people with type 2 diabetes.

However, the long-term safety and efficacy of the Atkins Diet are still being studied, and some research has raised concerns about the potential health problems linked with high-fat diets. Before beginning the Atkins Diet, like with any other diet, it is critical to check with a healthcare physician.

Furthermore, the Atkins Diet has been shown to improve other health indices such as blood pressure, triglyceride levels, and HDL cholesterol levels. A meta-analysis of 17 randomized controlled studies published in 2018 showed that low-carbohydrate diets, including the Atkins Diet, were more successful than low-fat diets in lowering blood pressure and triglyceride levels.

The Atkins Diet has also been examined for its possible advantages in the treatment of neurological illnesses such as epilepsy and Alzheimer's. Ketones created during the ketosis process have been demonstrated to have neuroprotective properties and may enhance cognitive performance in people suffering from neurological disorders.

It is important to remember, however, that the Atkins Diet may not be ideal for everyone. During the first phase of the diet, some people may feel weariness, constipation, and poor breath. People with specific medical issues, such as renal disease, may need to reduce their protein consumption and should see a healthcare professional before beginning the Atkins Diet.

Overall, while the science behind the Atkins Diet is still advancing, it has yielded good outcomes in terms of weight reduction and metabolic health indicators. As with any diet, the Atkins Diet should be approached carefully and under the supervision of a healthcare expert.

Benefits of the Atkins Diet for Seniors

The Atkins Diet may provide various advantages to seniors, including:

Weight loss: As we age, our metabolism slows, making it more difficult to lose weight. The Atkins Diet's low-carbohydrate, high-protein strategy can help seniors lose weight and enhance their body composition.

Blood sugar control: Seniors are more likely than younger people to acquire type 2 diabetes, and the Atkins Diet's carbohydrate restriction can help control blood sugar levels and lower the risk of acquiring diabetes.

Cardiovascular health: Studies have indicated that the Atkins Diet improves lipid profile markers like triglycerides and HDL cholesterol, which are key indicators of cardiovascular health.

Brain health: The ketogenic state created by the Atkins Diet has been examined for its possible advantages in the management of neurological illnesses like Alzheimer's disease.

Improved energy and vitality: The Atkins Diet's emphasis on high-quality protein and healthy fats can give seniors sustained energy throughout the day and help them feel more alive.

It should be noted that the Atkins Diet may not be suitable for all seniors, particularly those with certain medical concerns or dietary limitations. Before beginning any new diet or fitness regimen, seniors should contact their healthcare physician.

In addition to the benefits listed above, the Atkins Diet may be beneficial for seniors who have certain health issues. As an example:

High blood pressure: The Atkins Diet's emphasis on limiting refined carbs while boosting intake of healthy fats and protein will help decrease blood pressure, which is especially beneficial for seniors who are predisposed to hypertension.

Arthritis: Some research suggests that a low-carbohydrate diet, such as the Atkins Diet, may be good for seniors suffering from osteoarthritis. The anti-inflammatory benefits of the diet can help lessen the pain and inflammation associated with arthritis.

Digestive problems: The Atkins Diet's emphasis on whole, unprocessed meals might be beneficial for seniors suffering from digestive problems such as bloating, gas, and constipation. The low-carbohydrate, high-fiber strategy of the diet helps support good digestion and regularity.

It should be noted that the Atkins Diet is not a one-size-fits-all strategy and may not be appropriate for everyone. Seniors should consult with their healthcare physician to see if the Atkins Diet is a good fit for their specific health concerns and objectives. To promote their general health and wellness, they should also ensure that they are fulfilling their nutrient needs and eating a range of full, nutrient-dense meals.

The Atkins Diet's Risks and Limitations for Seniors

While there are numerous possible benefits to the Atkins Diet for seniors, there are also certain hazards and restrictions to be aware of. These are some examples:

Nutrient deficiencies: Because the Atkins Diet is low in carbs, it might be difficult to achieve daily nutrient demands, especially for seniors who may have a lower appetite or difficulties eating. It's critical for seniors on the Atkins Diet to receive adequate vitamins, minerals, and fiber from nutrient-dense foods like vegetables, fruits, and whole grains.

Kidney function: The Atkins Diet's high protein consumption might place extra strain on the kidneys, which can be troublesome for seniors who already have kidney problems. Before beginning the Atkins Diet, seniors with renal disease or other kidney-related health issues should contact their healthcare physician.

Dehydration: The Atkins Diet's emphasis on protein and fat can contribute to dehydration, particularly in seniors who are already predisposed to dehydration. To be adequately hydrated, seniors on the Atkins Diet should consume lots of water and other hydrating drinks.

Adherence issues: The Atkins Diet can be difficult to stick to over time, especially for seniors who may have fewer food alternatives or trouble cooking. Seniors should collaborate with their healthcare physician and a qualified dietitian to develop a long-term food plan that suits their specific health needs and objectives.

While the Atkins Diet has been found in some trials to improve lipid indicators, other research has revealed that high-protein, high-fat diets may raise the risk of heart disease, particularly in seniors who may already have underlying cardiovascular difficulties. Seniors should consult with their healthcare physician to see whether the Atkins Diet is a good fit for them based on their own health history.

It is critical for seniors to consult with their healthcare physician and a qualified dietitian to decide whether the Atkins Diet is a good fit for their specific health requirements and objectives. Seniors should also keep a close eye on their health and well-being while on the diet and seek medical assistance if they encounter any negative side effects.

CHAPTER TWO

MODIFYING THE ATKINS DIET FOR SENIORS

Seniors' Specific Nutritional Needs

Seniors have different dietary requirements than younger individuals. Among these requirements are:

Adequate protein: As they age, seniors may require extra protein to promote muscle maintenance and repair. Protein is also necessary for immunological function and wound repair.

Increased fiber: To promote digestive health and prevent constipation, seniors may require extra fiber. Fiber-rich diets can also help decrease cholesterol and the risk of heart disease.

Sufficient hydration: Seniors may be more susceptible to dehydration owing to a diminished sensation of thirst or mobility issues. It is critical for seniors to drink adequate fluids throughout the day, including water and other hydrating liquids.

Adequate vitamin and mineral intake: Because of changes in their digestive system, seniors may have trouble absorbing some nutrients, such as vitamin B12 and vitamin D. As a result, they may need to take supplements or eat fortified meals to ensure they obtain enough of these vital elements.

Limit your salt intake: Seniors are more likely to develop high blood pressure, which can lead to heart disease and stroke. Blood pressure can be managed by limiting sodium consumption, avoiding processed and packaged meals, and cooking with herbs and spices instead of salt.

A balanced and diverse diet that includes a mix of fruits, vegetables, whole grains, lean meats, and healthy fats should be consumed by seniors. This can help ensure kids obtain all of the nutrients they require to maintain their health and well-being.

Overall, seniors should collaborate with a healthcare professional and a registered dietitian to develop a tailored meal plan that addresses their specific nutritional needs and health objectives.

In addition to the aforementioned dietary requirements, seniors may require some nutrients in greater quantities than younger people. These are some examples:

Calcium: Calcium is essential for seniors to maintain bone health and avoid osteoporosis. Dairy products, fortified plant-based milks, and leafy green vegetables are all good calcium sources.

Vitamin D: Because seniors may have difficulties manufacturing vitamin D in their skin from sunlight, they may need supplements or fortified meals to keep their bones strong and prevent falls.

Vitamin B12: Because of changes in the digestive tract, seniors may have trouble absorbing vitamin B12 from food. This vitamin is essential for nerve function and red blood cell formation. Meat, fish, eggs, and fortified meals are high in vitamin B12.

Potassium: Seniors may need additional potassium to help manage blood pressure and keep their hearts healthy. Bananas, oranges, tomatoes, leafy green vegetables, and beans are high in potassium.

Omega-3 fatty acids: Consuming extra omega-3 fatty acids may enhance seniors' cognitive and heart health. Fatty fish, such as salmon and tuna, as well as flaxseed, chia seeds, and walnuts, are high in omega-3s.

Seniors should eat nutrient-dense meals that include a range of vitamins, minerals, and other helpful components. Furthermore, seniors should strive to restrict their consumption of processed and refined foods, sugary beverages, and saturated and trans fats, which might raise the risk of chronic illnesses including heart disease, diabetes, and some malignancies.

Adapting the Atkins Diet for Seniors

While the Atkins Diet has been found to be beneficial for weight reduction and the improvement of some health concerns, it may not be suitable or safe for all seniors. As a result, it is critical to tailor the Atkins diet to the specific demands of older people.

The Atkins Diet can be modified for seniors in the following ways:

Carbohydrate consumption should be adjusted to: Seniors may require somewhat more carbs than younger people to meet energy demands and preserve muscular mass. As a result, increasing the quantity of carbs permitted on the Atkins Diet for seniors may be advantageous.

Increasing protein consumption: Seniors may need extra protein to maintain muscle mass and avoid muscle atrophy. It may be good for seniors to increase the quantity of protein permitted on the Atkins Diet while ensuring that protein sources are lean and nutrient-dense.

Incorporating nutrient-dense foods: As previously noted, seniors have special nutritional demands and may require more vitamins and minerals than younger people. To satisfy these requirements, the Atkins Diet for Seniors should include a range of nutrient-dense foods such as fruits, vegetables, whole grains, lean meats, and healthy fats.

Keeping hydrated: Seniors may be more susceptible to dehydration, which can lead to a range of health problems. It is critical that seniors on the Atkins Diet drink adequate fluids throughout the day and consume hydrating meals like fruits and vegetables.

Collaboration with a healthcare professional: Before beginning any diet, seniors should check with their healthcare practitioner to confirm that it is safe and appropriate for their specific needs and health concerns. A healthcare practitioner can also assist elders in customizing the Atkins Diet to match their specific needs and making any required changes.

Calculating Your Daily Carbohydrate Intake

Following the Atkins Diet requires you to calculate your daily carbohydrate consumption. The idea is to decrease your daily carbohydrate intake while boosting your intake of protein and healthy fats.

Follow these procedures to calculate your daily carbohydrate consumption on the Atkins Diet:

Determine your daily calorie requirements: The first step is to figure out how many calories you need each day to stay at the same weight. This can be accomplished through the use of a calorie calculator or by speaking with a healthcare expert.

Calculate your carbohydrate intake: The amount of carbs you consume each day on the Atkins Diet is determined by the phase of the diet you are on. Carbohydrate consumption is restricted to 20–25 grams per day during the initial phase, termed the "induction" phase. Carbohydrate consumption can be gradually raised in succeeding periods.

Calculate your daily carbohydrate consumption: Once you've determined your daily calorie requirements and ideal carbohydrate intake, you can figure out what proportion of your daily calories should come from carbs. For example, if you eat 1,500 calories per day and limit your carbohydrate intake to 20 grams per day, you will get 80 calories from carbs. Divide the total calories from carbs by the total calories ingested and multiply by 100 to get the percentage. The proportion in this scenario would be 5.3%.

Track your carbohydrate consumption: Once you've decided your daily carbohydrate intake, it's critical to keep track of it to ensure you're remaining under your daily limit. This can be accomplished through the use of a meal diary or a smartphone app that records macronutrient consumption.

It's crucial to remember that calculating your daily carbohydrate consumption is only one part of the Atkins Diet. It is also critical to consume a range of nutrient-dense meals, remain hydrated, and collaborate with a healthcare practitioner to make any required dietary changes depending on your unique needs and health concerns.

On the Atkins Diet, here's an example of how to calculate your daily carbohydrate intake:

Assume you are a 65-year-old lady weighing 160 pounds and standing 5'6" tall. You decide that you need 1,500 calories per day to maintain your current weight based on your exercise level and other considerations.

You decide to limit your carbohydrate consumption to 20 grams per day during the initial "induction" phase of the Atkins Diet. Follow these procedures to calculate the percentage of your daily calories that should come from carbohydrates:

Determine the number of calories in 20 grams of carbs: Because each gram of carbohydrates contains 4 calories, 20 grams of carbohydrates equals 80 calories.

Calculate the percentage of calories that should be derived from carbohydrates. Divide the calories from carbs by your entire daily calorie requirements and multiply by 100. In this scenario, the computation would be as follows:

80 carbohydrate calories x 1,500 total daily calories x 100 = 5.3%

During the Atkins Diet's induction phase, you should aim to take no more than 5.3% of your daily calories from carbs, or around 20 grams per day. You would progressively increase your carbohydrate consumption as you progressed through the diet phases while remaining under your recommended daily limit.

Diet tips that make it easier to stick to

Here are some pointers to help you stick to the Atkins Diet:

Meal planning: Plan your meals and snacks ahead of time to ensure you remain under your daily carbohydrate allowance. When you're hungry and short on time, this can also help you resist the urge to go for high-carb quick items.

Cooking in bulk: Make huge quantities of dishes and freeze them in individual servings. In the long term, this may save you time and energy while also ensuring that you always have a low-carb meal on hand when you need it.

Portion management is important, especially when eating high-carb meals like fruits, grains, and starchy vegetables. To ensure that you remain within your daily carbohydrate allowance, use measuring cups or a food scale.

Experiment with new meals: When you try new low-carb recipes and ingredients, the Atkins Diet can be delicious and rewarding. Look for cookbooks or websites that specialize in low-carb cooking.

Drink Water: Drink lots of water and other non-caloric liquids to feel full and content, as well as to prevent constipation, which can be a side effect of the low-carb diet.

Seek help: Seek help from family, friends, or a healthcare professional who can give direction and inspiration as you strive toward your Atkins Diet health objectives.

CHAPTER THREE

EATING ON THE ATKINS DIET

Meal preparation on the Atkins Diet

Meal preparation for the Atkins Diet entails selecting meals that are low in carbs and rich in protein and healthy fats. The idea is to restrict your carbohydrate consumption while still receiving enough nutrients and energy to feel satiated and invigorated.

Here are some Atkins Diet meal planning suggestions:

Protein-rich foods: Include lots of lean protein sources in your meals, such as chicken, fish, eggs, and tofu, to help you feel full and content.

Choose healthy fats such as avocado, almonds, seeds, and olive oil to help you satisfy your calorie demands while also supporting your overall health.

Include low-carb veggies: Choose non-starchy vegetables like leafy greens, broccoli, cauliflower, and peppers to acquire key vitamins and minerals while limiting your carbohydrate intake.

Avoid or restrict high-carb foods, such as bread, pasta, rice, and sugary snacks and sweets.

Make a plan: Plan your meals and snacks ahead of time to ensure you remain under your daily carbohydrate limit and acquire all the nutrients you require.

Keep track of your progress: Keep track of your weight, energy levels, and other health indicators to confirm that the Atkins Diet is working for you and improving your health.

Portion management is essential: Because even low-carb foods can be heavy in calories, it's critical to exercise portion control and prevent overeating.

Experiment with recipes: To keep your meals interesting and fulfilling, look for low-carb recipes and experiment with different flavor combinations and cooking techniques.

Drink Water: Drink lots of water throughout the day to keep hydrated and to aid digestion and metabolism.

Consider supplements: Seniors may have specific dietary requirements, so talk to your doctor or a qualified dietitian about whether calcium, vitamin D, or B12 supplements may be useful to you.

Seniors may cook tasty, enjoyable meals that fit their specific nutritional demands while also supporting their general health and well-being by following these ideas and guidelines.

Atkins Recipes for Seniors

Breakfast

Here are healthy and tasty low-carb recipes that are perfect for seniors following the Atkins Diet:

Grilled Salmon with Asparagus and Cauliflower Rice

Ingredients:

4 salmon fillets

1 lb asparagus

1 head cauliflower

2 cloves garlic, minced

1 lemon, sliced

3 tbsp olive oil

Salt and pepper to taste

Instructions:

Preheat grill to medium-high heat.

Cut the cauliflower into small florets and pulse in a food processor until it resembles rice.

In a large skillet, heat 1 tbsp of olive oil over medium heat. Add the minced garlic and cook for 1-2 minutes.

Add the cauliflower rice to the skillet and sauté until tender, about 5-7 minutes.

Toss the asparagus in 2 tbsp of olive oil and season with salt and pepper. Grill for 5-7 minutes, turning occasionally.

Season the salmon with salt and pepper and grill for 5-7 minutes per side.

Serve the salmon with the grilled asparagus, cauliflower rice, and lemon slices.

Nutritional Information (per serving):

Calories: 397

Fat: 23g

Protein: 39g

Carbohydrates: 10g

Fiber: 5g

Chicken Broccoli Alfredo

Ingredients:

4 chicken breasts, sliced into thin strips

1 head broccoli, chopped

2 cloves garlic, minced

1 cup heavy cream

1/2 cup grated Parmesan cheese

2 tbsp butter

Salt and pepper to taste

Instructions:

In a large skillet, heat 2 tbsp of butter over medium heat. Add the minced garlic and cook for 1-2 minutes.

Add the chicken strips to the skillet and cook until browned and cooked through, about 5-7 minutes.

Add the chopped broccoli to the skillet and cook for an additional 3-4 minutes.

Add the heavy cream and Parmesan cheese to the skillet and stir until the sauce is thickened and creamy.

Season with salt and pepper to taste.

Serve hot.

Nutritional Information (per serving):

Calories: 426

Fat: 29g

Protein: 34g

Carbohydrates: 9g

Fiber: 3g

Zucchini Noodle Lasagna

Ingredients:

2 large zucchini, spiralized

1 lb ground beef

1 cup low-carb tomato sauce

1 cup ricotta cheese

1 cup shredded mozzarella cheese

2 cloves garlic, minced

Salt and pepper to taste

Instructions:

Preheat oven to 375°F.

In a large skillet, cook the ground beef over medium heat until browned and cooked through.

Add the minced garlic and tomato sauce to the skillet and cook for 2-3 minutes.

In a greased 9x13 inch baking dish, layer the zucchini noodles, meat sauce, ricotta cheese, and shredded mozzarella cheese.

Repeat until all ingredients are used up, ending with a layer of mozzarella cheese on top.

Cover the baking dish with foil and bake for 30 minutes.

Remove the foil and bake for an additional 10-15 minutes until the cheese is golden brown.

Serve hot.

Nutritional Information (per serving):

Calories: 366

Fat: 23g / Protein: 31g

Carbohydrates: 9g / Fiber: 2g

Grilled Salmon with Asparagus

Ingredients:

4 salmon fillets (4-6 ounces each)

1 pound asparagus, trimmed

2 tablespoons olive oil

Salt and pepper to taste

Lemon wedges for serving

Instructions:

Preheat a grill to medium-high heat.

Season the salmon fillets with salt and pepper.

Toss the asparagus with 1 tablespoon of olive oil and season with salt and pepper.

Grill the salmon fillets for 5-7 minutes per side, or until cooked through.

Grill the asparagus for 5-7 minutes, or until tender.

Drizzle the salmon and asparagus with the remaining olive oil and serve with lemon wedges.

Nutrition Information:

Calories: 386

Fat: 23g

Protein: 39g

Carbohydrates: 5g

Fiber: 3g

Net Carbs: 2g

Greek Salad with Grilled Chicken

Ingredients:

4 boneless, skinless chicken breasts

4 cups mixed greens

1 cucumber, chopped

1/2 red onion, sliced

1/2 cup cherry tomatoes, halved

1/4 cup kalamata olives, sliced

1/4 cup crumbled feta cheese

2 tablespoons olive oil

2 tablespoons red wine vinegar

Salt and pepper to taste

Instructions:

Preheat a grill to medium-high heat.

Season the chicken breasts with salt and pepper.

Grill the chicken for 5-7 minutes per side, or until cooked through.

In a large bowl, combine the mixed greens, cucumber, red onion, cherry tomatoes, and kalamata olives.

In a small bowl, whisk together the olive oil, red wine vinegar, salt, and pepper to make the dressing.

Slice the grilled chicken and add it to the salad.

Drizzle the salad with the dressing and sprinkle with crumbled feta cheese.

Nutrition Information:

Calories: 399

Fat: 21g

Protein: 42g

Carbohydrates: 10g

Fiber: 3g

Net Carbs: 7g

Zucchini Noodles with Meat Sauce

Ingredients:

4 medium zucchini, spiralized

1 pound ground beef

1 can (14 ounces) diced tomatoes

2 cloves garlic, minced

1 tablespoon olive oil

1 teaspoon dried basil

1/2 teaspoon dried oregano

Salt and pepper to taste

Grated Parmesan cheese for serving

Instructions:

Heat the olive oil in a large skillet over medium-high heat.

Add the ground beef and cook, breaking it up with a wooden spoon, until browned.

Add the garlic, basil, oregano, salt, and pepper to the skillet and cook for 1-2 minutes, or until fragrant.

Add the diced tomatoes and their juice to the skillet and bring to a simmer.

Reduce the heat to low and let the sauce simmer for 10-15 minutes, or until thickened.

While the sauce is cooking, spiralize the zucchini into noodles.

Bring a pot of salted water to a boil and cook the zucchini noodles for 1-2 minutes, or until tender.

Drain the noodles and divide

Once the sauce is heated through, add the zucchini noodles to the skillet and toss to combine with the sauce.

Cook for an additional 2-3 minutes, or until the zucchini noodles are tender but still slightly firm.

Divide the zucchini noodles and meat sauce evenly between four serving bowls.

Garnish each serving with a sprinkle of fresh parsley and a few shavings of Parmesan cheese.

Serve hot and enjoy!

Nutritional information per serving:

Calories: 282

Protein: 24g

Fat: 16g / Carbohydrates: 11g / Fiber: 3g

Sugar: 7g / Sodium: 435mg

Grilled Salmon with Mango Salsa

Ingredients:

4 salmon fillets

1 mango, peeled and diced

1 small red onion, diced

1 jalapeno pepper, seeded and minced

1 lime, juiced

2 tbsp fresh cilantro, chopped

Salt and pepper

Cooking spray

Instructions:

Preheat grill to medium-high heat.

Season salmon fillets with salt and pepper.

Spray the grill grates with cooking spray.

Grill salmon fillets for 4-5 minutes per side, or until cooked through.

While the salmon is cooking, make the mango salsa by combining diced mango, red onion, jalapeno pepper, lime juice, and cilantro in a bowl.

Serve the grilled salmon topped with the mango salsa.

Enjoy!

Nutritional information per serving:

Calories: 315

Protein: 37g

Fat: 15g

Carbohydrates: 11g

Fiber: 2g

Sugar: 8g

Sodium: 68mg

Quinoa Salad with Roasted Vegetables

Ingredients:

1 cup quinoa

2 cups water

1 red bell pepper, seeded and chopped

1 zucchini, chopped

1 yellow squash, chopped

1 small red onion, chopped

1 tbsp olive oil

2 tbsp balsamic vinegar

1 tsp honey

Salt and pepper

1/4 cup crumbled feta cheese

2 tbsp chopped fresh parsley

Instructions:

Preheat oven to 400°F.

Rinse quinoa under running water and add it to a pot with water. Bring to a boil, reduce heat to low, and simmer for 15-20 minutes or until the quinoa is tender.

While the quinoa is cooking, toss the chopped vegetables in olive oil and season with salt and pepper.

Spread the vegetables on a baking sheet and roast in the preheated oven for 20-25 minutes, or until tender and slightly caramelized.

In a small bowl, whisk together balsamic vinegar, honey, salt, and pepper.

In a large bowl, combine cooked quinoa, roasted vegetables, feta cheese, and parsley.

Drizzle the balsamic dressing over the quinoa salad and toss to combine.

Serve and enjoy!

Nutritional information per serving:

Calories: 300

Protein: 10g

Fat: 10g

Carbohydrates: 44g

Fiber: 7g

Sugar: 9g

Sodium: 175mg

Turkey and Vegetable Stir-Fry

Ingredients:

1 lb ground turkey

1 small onion, chopped

1 red bell pepper, chopped

2 cups broccoli florets

2 cups sliced mushrooms

1 tbsp olive oil

2 garlic cloves, minced

1 tsp ginger, minced

1/4 cup soy sauce

2 tbsp rice vinegar

2 tbsp honey

Salt and pepper

Instructions:

In a large skillet, heat olive oil over medium-high heat.

Add onion and cook for 2-3 minutes or until translucent.

Add ground turkey and cook for 5-6 minutes or until browned and cooked through.

Add broccoli, red bell pepper, and mushrooms to the skillet and cook for an additional 4-Minute.

Add the zucchini, bell pepper, and broccoli to the skillet. Stir-fry for 2-3 minutes or until the vegetables are tender-crisp.

Return the turkey to the skillet and stir-fry for an additional minute.

In a small bowl, whisk together the soy sauce, rice vinegar, garlic, and ginger. Pour the sauce over the stir-fry and stir to coat.

Serve hot with brown rice or quinoa, if desired.

Nutritional Information (per serving):

Calories: 282

Protein: 30g

Carbohydrates: 18g

Fat: 10g

Fiber: 5g

Sodium: 630mg

Grilled Salmon with Avocado Salsa

Ingredients:

4 salmon fillets

1 avocado, diced

1/2 red onion, diced

1 jalapeno pepper, seeded and minced

1 lime, juiced

2 tablespoons chopped cilantro

Salt and pepper, to taste

Instructions:

Preheat grill to medium-high heat.

Season the salmon fillets with salt and pepper.

Grill the salmon for 4-5 minutes per side or until cooked through.

While the salmon is cooking, prepare the avocado salsa by combining the diced avocado, red onion, jalapeno pepper, lime juice, cilantro, and a pinch of salt in a small bowl.

Top each salmon fillet with the avocado salsa.

Serve hot with a side of steamed vegetables or a mixed greens salad.

Nutritional Information (per serving):

Calories: 345

Protein: 30g

Carbohydrates: 10g

Fat: 22g

Fiber: 7g

Sodium: 110mg

Note: Nutritional information may vary depending on the specific ingredients and brands used.

Recipes for Lunch

Here are the healthy and delicious lunch recipes:

Quinoa and Vegetable Salad

Ingredients:

1 cup quinoa

2 cups water

1 red bell pepper, chopped

1 yellow bell pepper, chopped

1 cucumber, chopped

1 avocado, diced

1/4 cup chopped fresh cilantro

1/4 cup olive oil

2 tablespoons lime juice

Salt and pepper to taste

Instructions:

Rinse the quinoa thoroughly and drain.

In a medium saucepan, bring the water to a boil. Add the quinoa and reduce the heat to low. Cover and simmer for 15-20 minutes, or until the quinoa is tender and the water has been absorbed.

In a large bowl, combine the cooked quinoa, bell peppers, cucumber, avocado, and cilantro.

In a small bowl, whisk together the olive oil, lime juice, salt, and pepper.

Drizzle the dressing over the salad and toss gently to combine.

Nutritional information per serving (makes 4 servings):

Calories: 332

Protein: 7g

Fat: 22g

Carbohydrates: 29g

Fiber: 8g

Chickpea and Sweet Potato Stew

Ingredients:

1 tablespoon olive oil

1 onion, chopped

2 cloves garlic, minced

1 teaspoon ground cumin

1 teaspoon smoked paprika

1/4 teaspoon cayenne pepper

2 cups vegetable broth

1 can (14 ounces) diced tomatoes

2 sweet potatoes, peeled and cubed

1 can (14 ounces) chickpeas, drained and rinsed

1 cup chopped kale

Salt and pepper to taste

Instructions:

In a large pot, heat the olive oil over medium heat. Add the onion and garlic and sauté until the onion is translucent.

Add the cumin, smoked paprika, and cayenne pepper and stir to combine.

Add the vegetable broth, diced tomatoes, and sweet potatoes. Bring to a simmer and cook for 20 minutes, or until the sweet potatoes are tender.

Add the chickpeas and kale and simmer for another 5 minutes, or until the kale is wilted.

Season with salt and pepper to taste.

Nutritional information per serving (makes 4 servings):

Calories: 256 / Protein: 8g

Fat: 4g / Carbohydrates: 49g / Fiber: 11g

Tuna Salad with Greek Yogurt

Ingredients:

1 can (5 ounces) tuna, drained

1/4 cup plain Greek yogurt

1 tablespoon Dijon mustard

1 stalk celery, finely chopped

1/4 cup finely chopped red onion

2 tablespoons chopped fresh parsley

Salt and pepper to taste

4 cups mixed salad greens

Instructions:

In a medium bowl, mix together the tuna, Greek yogurt, Dijon mustard, celery, red onion, parsley, salt, and pepper.

Divide the mixed salad greens between four plates.

Top each plate of greens with a quarter of the tuna salad.

Nutritional information per serving (makes 4 servings):

Calories: 101 / Protein: 12g

Fat: 3g / Carbohydrates: 6g / Fiber: 2g

Grilled Chicken and Quinoa Salad:

Ingredients:

1 cup cooked quinoa

2 cups mixed greens

1 grilled chicken breast, sliced

1/4 cup crumbled feta cheese

1/4 cup sliced almonds

1/4 cup dried cranberries

2 tablespoons olive oil

1 tablespoon balsamic vinegar

Salt and pepper to taste

Instructions:

In a large bowl, combine the cooked quinoa and mixed greens.

Top with sliced grilled chicken, crumbled feta cheese, sliced almonds, and dried cranberries.

In a small bowl, whisk together the olive oil and balsamic vinegar. Season with salt and pepper to taste.

Drizzle the dressing over the salad and toss to combine.

Serve immediately.

Nutritional Information (per serving):

Calories: 485

Protein: 34g

Fat: 27g

Carbohydrates: 29g

Fiber: 5g

Sugar: 11g

Tuna Avocado Lettuce Wraps:

Ingredients:

1 can tuna, drained

1 avocado, diced

1/4 cup diced red onion

1/4 cup diced celery

1 tablespoon lemon juice

Salt and pepper to taste

4 large lettuce leaves

Instructions:

In a bowl, combine the drained tuna, diced avocado, red onion, and celery.

Add lemon juice and season with salt and pepper to taste.

Place a spoonful of the tuna mixture onto each lettuce leaf.

Roll up the lettuce leaves to form wraps.

Serve immediately.

Nutritional Information (per serving):

Calories: 205

Protein: 16g

Fat: 13g

Carbohydrates: 9g

Fiber: 5g

Sugar: 2g

Chickpea and Veggie Bowl:

Ingredients:

1 cup cooked brown rice

1 cup cooked chickpeas

1 cup roasted mixed vegetables (such as broccoli, carrots, and bell peppers)

1/4 cup crumbled feta cheese

1 tablespoon olive oil

1 tablespoon lemon juice

Salt and pepper to taste

Instructions:

In a bowl, combine the cooked brown rice, cooked chickpeas, and roasted mixed vegetables.

Top with crumbled feta cheese.

In a small bowl, whisk together the olive oil and lemon juice. Season with salt and pepper to taste.

Drizzle the dressing over the bowl and toss to combine.

Serve immediately.

Nutritional Information (per serving):

Calories: 448

Protein: 15g

Fat: 15g

Carbohydrates: 63g

Fiber: 10g

Sugar: 4g

Grilled Chicken Salad:

Ingredients:

4 oz grilled chicken breast

2 cups mixed greens

1/4 cup cherry tomatoes, halved

1/4 cup sliced cucumber

1/4 cup sliced red onion

1/4 cup sliced carrots

2 tbsp balsamic vinaigrette

Instructions:

Preheat grill to medium heat.

Season chicken with salt and pepper.

Grill chicken for 4-5 minutes per side until cooked through.

Let chicken rest for 5 minutes and then slice into strips.

In a large bowl, combine mixed greens, cherry tomatoes, cucumber, red onion, and carrots.

Top salad with sliced chicken.

Drizzle with balsamic vinaigrette and toss to combine.

Nutrition information:

Calories: 291

Protein: 28g

Fat: 12g

Carbohydrates: 15g

Fiber: 4g

Quinoa and Black Bean Bowl:

Ingredients:

1 cup cooked quinoa

1/2 cup black beans, rinsed and drained

1/2 avocado, diced

1/4 cup diced red onion

1/4 cup diced red bell pepper

1/4 cup chopped cilantro

2 tbsp lime juice

1 tbsp olive oil

Salt and pepper to taste

Instructions:

In a large bowl, combine cooked quinoa, black beans, avocado, red onion, red bell pepper, and cilantro.

In a separate small bowl, whisk together lime juice, olive oil, salt, and pepper.

Drizzle dressing over the quinoa and black bean mixture and toss to combine.

Nutrition information:

Calories: 399

Protein: 13g

Fat: 20g

Carbohydrates: 43g

Fiber: 13g

Tuna and Egg Salad:

Ingredients:

1 can tuna, drained

2 hard-boiled eggs, chopped

1/4 cup chopped celery

1/4 cup chopped red onion

2 tbsp chopped parsley

2 tbsp lemon juice

2 tbsp olive oil

Salt and pepper to taste

Instructions:

In a large bowl, combine tuna, chopped hard-boiled eggs, celery, red onion, and parsley.

In a separate small bowl, whisk together lemon juice, olive oil, salt, and pepper.

Drizzle dressing over the tuna and egg mixture and toss to combine.

Nutrition information:

Calories: 304

Protein: 29g

Fat: 18g

Carbohydrates: 4g

Fiber: 1g

Recipes for Dinner

Grilled Lemon Herb Chicken

Ingredients:

4 boneless, skinless chicken breasts

2 tablespoons olive oil

2 tablespoons chopped fresh parsley

2 tablespoons chopped fresh rosemary

1 tablespoon chopped fresh thyme

Juice of 1 lemon

Salt and black pepper to taste

Instructions:

Preheat grill to medium-high heat.

In a small bowl, mix together olive oil, parsley, rosemary, thyme, lemon juice, salt, and pepper.

Place chicken breasts in a resealable plastic bag and pour the marinade over them. Seal the bag and massage the chicken to coat evenly.

Allow the chicken to marinate for at least 30 minutes, or overnight for best results.

Grill the chicken for 5-6 minutes per side, or until the internal temperature reaches 165°F.

Remove the chicken from the grill and let it rest for 5 minutes before serving.

Nutritional Information per serving:

Calories: 190

Protein: 27g

Fat: 8g

Carbohydrates: 0g

Fiber: 0g

Sugar: 0g

Sodium: 115mg

Baked Salmon with Asparagus

Ingredients:

4 salmon fillets

1 pound asparagus, trimmed

2 tablespoons olive oil

2 cloves garlic, minced

1 tablespoon chopped fresh parsley

Salt and black pepper to taste

Instructions:

Preheat the oven to 400°F.

Line a baking sheet with parchment paper.

In a small bowl, mix together olive oil, garlic, parsley, salt, and pepper.

Place the salmon fillets on the prepared baking sheet.

Drizzle the oil mixture over the salmon fillets.

Place the asparagus on the baking sheet around the salmon fillets.

Bake in the preheated oven for 12-15 minutes or until the salmon is cooked through and the asparagus is tender.

Nutritional Information per serving:

Calories: 390

Protein: 34g

Fat: 25g

Carbohydrates: 6g

Fiber: 3g

Sugar: 3g

Sodium: 190mg

Grilled Salmon with Asparagus

Ingredients:

4 salmon fillets

1 pound asparagus

1 tablespoon olive oil

1 clove garlic, minced

1 tablespoon lemon juice

Salt and black pepper to taste

Instructions:

Preheat the grill to medium-high heat.

Rinse the asparagus and trim off the woody ends.

In a small bowl, whisk together the olive oil, garlic, lemon juice, salt, and black pepper.

Brush the salmon fillets and asparagus with the olive oil mixture.

Place the salmon fillets and asparagus on the grill and cook for about 5-7 minutes on each side or until the salmon is cooked through and the asparagus is tender.

Serve hot.

Nutrition Information (per serving):

Calories: 348 kcal

Fat: 23g

Protein: 30g

Carbohydrates: 6g

Fiber: 3g

Baked Chicken with Broccoli and Cheese

Ingredients:

4 boneless, skinless chicken breasts

1 head of broccoli, cut into florets

1 cup shredded cheddar cheese

1/4 cup mayonnaise

2 tablespoons Dijon mustard

1 clove garlic, minced

Salt and black pepper to taste

Instructions:

Preheat the oven to 375°F.

Season the chicken breasts with salt and black pepper.

Arrange the chicken breasts in a baking dish.

In a small bowl, whisk together the mayonnaise, Dijon mustard, garlic, salt, and black pepper.

Spread the mayonnaise mixture over the chicken breasts.

Top the chicken breasts with the broccoli florets and shredded cheddar cheese.

Bake in the oven for 25-30 minutes or until the chicken is cooked through and the cheese is melted and bubbly.

Serve hot.

Nutrition Information (per serving):

Calories: 445 kcal

Fat: 27g

Protein: 41g

Carbohydrates: 7g

Fiber: 3g

Beef and Broccoli Stir-Fry

Ingredients:

1 pound flank steak, thinly sliced

2 cups broccoli florets

1 bell pepper, sliced

1 onion, sliced

2 cloves garlic, minced

1 tablespoon ginger, minced

2 tablespoons soy sauce

2 tablespoons olive oil

Salt and black pepper to taste

Instructions:

Heat the olive oil in a wok or large skillet over high heat.

Add the garlic and ginger and cook for 30 seconds or until fragrant.

Add the sliced beef and stir-fry for 2-3 minutes or until browned.

Add the broccoli florets, bell pepper, and onion and stir-fry for another 3-4 minutes or until the vegetables are tender-crisp.

Drizzle the soy sauce over the stir-fry and toss to combine.

Season with salt and black pepper to taste.

Serve hot.

Nutrition Information (per serving):

Calories: 355 kcal

Fat: 19g

Protein: 32g

Carbohydrates: 10g

Fiber: 3g

Grilled Salmon with Avocado Salsa

Ingredients:

4 salmon fillets

2 ripe avocados, diced

1 small red onion, diced

1 small jalapeno, seeded and finely chopped

2 tbsp chopped fresh cilantro

Juice of 1 lime

Salt and pepper to taste

Instructions:

Preheat grill to medium-high heat.

Season salmon fillets with salt and pepper.

Grill salmon for 6-8 minutes per side or until cooked through.

Meanwhile, in a medium bowl, combine diced avocados, red onion, jalapeno, cilantro, lime juice, salt, and pepper.

Serve salmon with avocado salsa on top.

Nutritional information (per serving):

Calories: 361

Protein: 34g

Fat: 23g

Carbohydrates: 9g

Fiber: 6g

Spicy Shrimp Stir-Fry

Ingredients:

1 lb shrimp, peeled and deveined

1 red bell pepper, sliced

1 yellow bell pepper, sliced

1 small onion, sliced

1 jalapeno pepper, seeded and chopped

2 cloves garlic, minced

2 tbsp olive oil

2 tbsp soy sauce

1 tbsp honey

1 tsp cornstarch

Salt and pepper to taste

Instructions:

In a small bowl, whisk together soy sauce, honey, cornstarch, and 1/4 cup of water.

Heat olive oil in a large skillet over medium-high heat.

Add sliced onions, bell peppers, jalapeno, and garlic to the skillet and sauté for 3-4 minutes until softened.

Add shrimp to the skillet and cook until pink, about 2-3 minutes.

Pour the soy sauce mixture over the shrimp and vegetables, and stir well to combine.

Cook for an additional 2-3 minutes until the sauce thickens.

Serve hot with brown rice or quinoa.

Nutritional information (per serving):

Calories: 270

Protein: 25g

Fat: 10g

Carbohydrates: 20g

Fiber: 3g

Grilled Chicken with Roasted Vegetables

Ingredients:

4 boneless, skinless chicken breasts

2 bell peppers, seeded and sliced

2 zucchinis, sliced

1 red onion, sliced

1/4 cup olive oil

2 tbsp balsamic vinegar

2 cloves garlic, minced

Salt and pepper to taste

Instructions:

Preheat grill to medium-high heat.

In a small bowl, whisk together olive oil, balsamic vinegar, garlic, salt, and pepper.

Brush the chicken breasts with the olive oil mixture.

Grill chicken for 5-7 minutes per side or until cooked through.

Meanwhile, preheat oven to 425°F.

Spread sliced vegetables on a baking sheet and drizzle with remaining olive oil mixture.

Roast vegetables in the oven for 15-20 minutes or until tender.

Serve chicken with roasted vegetables on the side.

Nutritional information (per serving):

Calories: 346

Protein: 38g / Fat: 16g

Carbohydrates: 12g / Fiber: 3g

Garlic Ginger Baked Salmon

Ingredients:

4 salmon fillets

2 cloves garlic, minced

1 tablespoon grated ginger

1 tablespoon olive oil

1 tablespoon low-sodium soy sauce

1 tablespoon honey

1 tablespoon rice vinegar

Salt and pepper to taste

Lemon wedges for serving

Instructions:

Preheat the oven to 400°F (200°C).

In a small bowl, mix together the garlic, ginger, olive oil, soy sauce, honey, rice vinegar, salt, and pepper.

Place the salmon fillets on a baking sheet lined with parchment paper.

Spoon the garlic ginger sauce over the salmon fillets.

Bake the salmon for 12-15 minutes, or until the salmon is cooked through.

Serve with lemon wedges.

Nutritional Information per serving:

Calories: 308kcal

Carbohydrates: 6g

Protein: 33g

Fat: 17g

Saturated Fat: 3g

Cholesterol: 87mg

Sodium: 331mg

Potassium: 807mg

Fiber: 0g

Sugar: 5g

Vitamin A: 84IU

Vitamin C: 1mg

Calcium: 22mg

Iron: 2mg

Grilled Chicken and Vegetables Skewers

Ingredients:

4 chicken breasts, cut into bite-sized pieces

1 zucchini, cut into rounds

1 red bell pepper, cut into squares

1 yellow bell pepper, cut into squares

1 red onion, cut into wedges

1/4 cup olive oil

1 tablespoon balsamic vinegar

2 cloves garlic, minced

1 teaspoon dried oregano

Salt and pepper to taste

Wooden skewers

Instructions:

In a large bowl, whisk together the olive oil, balsamic vinegar, garlic, oregano, salt, and pepper.

Add the chicken pieces to the bowl and toss to coat.

Thread the marinated chicken and vegetables onto wooden skewers.

Heat a grill pan or outdoor grill to medium-high heat.

Place the skewers on the grill and cook for 8-10 minutes, flipping once, until the chicken is cooked through and the vegetables are tender.

Serve hot.

Nutritional Information per serving:

Calories: 270kcal

Carbohydrates: 9g

Protein: 29g

Fat: 14g

Saturated Fat: 2g

Cholesterol: 87mg

Sodium: 97mg

Potassium: 788mg

Fiber: 2g

Sugar: 5g

Vitamin A: 1789IU

Vitamin C: 100mg

Calcium: 32mg / Iron: 2mg

Stuffed Portobello Mushrooms

Ingredients:

4 large portobello mushroom caps

1/2 cup chopped onion

1/2 cup chopped red bell pepper

1/2 cup chopped zucchini

1/2 cup chopped yellow squash

2 cloves garlic, minced

1/2 teaspoon dried basil

1/2 teaspoon dried oregano

1/2 teaspoon salt

1/4 teaspoon black pepper

1/4 cup grated Parmesan cheese

1/4 cup chopped fresh parsley

1/4 cup shredded part-skim mozzarella cheese

Instructions:

Preheat the oven to 400°F (200°C).

Remove the stems from the mushrooms and clean the caps.

In a large skillet, sauté the onion, red bell pepper, zucchini, yellow squash, and garlic until the vegetables are tender, about 5 minutes.

Add the basil, oregano, salt, and black pepper to the skillet and stir to combine.

Remove the skillet from the heat and stir in the Parmesan cheese and parsley.

Divide the vegetable mixture evenly among the mushroom caps.

Place the stuffed mushrooms in a baking dish and bake for 20 minutes.

Sprinkle the mozzarella cheese over the top of the mushrooms and bake for an additional 5-7 minutes, until the cheese is melted and bubbly.

Remove the mushrooms from the oven and let cool for a few minutes before serving.

Nutritional Information:

Calories: 120

Fat: 5g

Protein: 11g

Carbohydrates: 12g

Fiber: 4g

Apple Slices with Almond Butter and Cinnamon

Ingredients:

1 medium apple, cored and sliced

2 tablespoons almond butter

1/4 teaspoon ground cinnamon

Instructions:

Arrange the apple slices on a plate or platter.

In a small bowl, mix the almond butter and cinnamon until well combined.

Dip the apple slices into the almond butter mixture and enjoy!

Nutritional Information (per serving):

Calories: 214

Fat: 14g

Carbohydrates: 20g

Fiber: 5g

Protein: 5g

Greek Yogurt with Berries and Honey

Ingredients:

1/2 cup plain Greek yogurt

1/2 cup mixed berries (such as strawberries, blueberries, and raspberries)

1 tablespoon honey

Instructions:

In a small bowl, mix the Greek yogurt and mixed berries until well combined.

Drizzle with honey and enjoy!

Nutritional Information (per serving):

Calories: 128

Fat: 0g

Carbohydrates: 21g

Fiber: 2g

Protein: 11g

Recipes for Snacks

here are the healthy snack recipes:

Greek Yogurt and Berry Parfait:

Ingredients:

1 cup plain Greek yogurt

1/2 cup mixed berries (such as strawberries, blueberries, and raspberries)

1 tablespoon honey

1/4 cup granola

Instructions:

In a small bowl, mix the Greek yogurt and honey together.

Layer the yogurt mixture, mixed berries, and granola in a parfait glass.

Serve immediately.

Nutritional Information:

Calories: 230

Protein: 18g

Carbohydrates: 31g

Fat: 5g / Fiber: 4g

Veggie Sticks with Hummus:

Ingredients:

1 medium carrot, peeled and cut into sticks

1 medium cucumber, cut into sticks

1 medium bell pepper, cut into strips

1/4 cup hummus

Instructions:

Arrange the vegetable sticks on a plate.

Serve with hummus for dipping.

Nutritional Information:

Calories: 120

Protein: 4g

Carbohydrates: 18g

Fat: 4g

Fiber: 7g

Apple Slices with Almond Butter:

Ingredients:

1 medium apple, sliced

2 tablespoons almond butter

Instructions:

Spread the almond butter on the apple slices.

Serve immediately.

Nutritional Information:

Calories: 210

Protein: 5g

Carbohydrates: 26g

Fat: 11g

Fiber: 5g

Apple Nachos

Ingredients:

1 apple, sliced

1 tbsp almond butter

1 tbsp dark chocolate chips

1 tbsp unsweetened shredded coconut

Instructions:

Arrange apple slices on a plate.

Melt almond butter and drizzle over the apple slices.

Sprinkle with chocolate chips and shredded coconut.

Serve and enjoy!

Nutritional information (per serving):

Calories: 198

Fat: 13g

Carbohydrates: 20g

Fiber: 6g

Protein: 3g

Roasted Chickpeas

Ingredients:

1 can (15 oz) chickpeas, drained and rinsed

1 tbsp olive oil

1 tsp garlic powder

1 tsp cumin

1 tsp paprika

Salt and pepper to taste

Instructions:

Preheat oven to 400°F.

Dry chickpeas with a paper towel.

In a bowl, mix chickpeas, olive oil, garlic powder, cumin, paprika, salt, and pepper until well combined.

Spread the mixture evenly on a baking sheet.

Roast in the oven for 20-25 minutes, or until chickpeas are crispy.

Serve and enjoy!

Nutritional information (per serving):

Calories: 167

Fat: 6g

Carbohydrates: 21g

Fiber: 6g

Protein: 7g

Cucumber Hummus Bites

Ingredients:

1 cucumber, sliced

1/4 cup hummus

Cherry tomatoes, halved

Fresh parsley or cilantro, chopped

Instructions:

Arrange cucumber slices on a plate.

Top each slice with a dollop of hummus.

Add a cherry tomato half on top of the hummus.

Sprinkle with chopped parsley or cilantro.

Serve and enjoy!

Nutritional information (per serving):

Calories: 64

Fat: 3g

Carbohydrates: 9g

Fiber: 2g

Protein: 2g

Greek Yogurt Dip:

Ingredients:

1 cup plain Greek yogurt

1 tbsp fresh dill, chopped

1 tbsp fresh parsley, chopped

1 tbsp fresh chives, chopped

1 clove garlic, minced

1/4 tsp salt

Freshly ground black pepper, to taste

Instructions:

In a bowl, mix together Greek yogurt, dill, parsley, chives, garlic, salt, and black pepper.

Chill in the refrigerator for at least 30 minutes to allow flavors to meld.

Serve with fresh vegetables or whole-grain crackers.

Nutritional information (per serving):

Calories: 69

Protein: 9g / Fat: 1g / Carbohydrates: 6g /

Fiber: 0g / Sugar: 4g/ Sodium: 189mg

Apple Slices with Almond Butter:

Ingredients:

1 medium apple, sliced

1 tbsp almond butter

1/4 tsp cinnamon

Instructions:

Spread almond butter on apple slices.

Sprinkle with cinnamon.

Nutritional information (per serving):

Calories: 148

Protein: 2g

Fat: 8g

Carbohydrates: 20g

Fiber: 4g

Sugar: 14g

Sodium: 2mg

Greek Yogurt and Fruit Parfait

Ingredients:

1 cup plain Greek yogurt

1 tablespoon honey

1/4 teaspoon vanilla extract

1/2 cup mixed berries (strawberries, blueberries, raspberries)

1/4 cup granola

Instructions:

In a small bowl, mix together the Greek yogurt, honey, and vanilla extract until well combined.

In a separate bowl, mix together the mixed berries.

In a serving glass or jar, layer the Greek yogurt mixture, followed by the mixed berries, and then the granola.

Repeat the layers until all ingredients are used up.

Top with a sprinkle of granola and a few fresh berries.

Chill in the refrigerator for at least 30 minutes to allow the flavors to meld together.

Serve and enjoy!

Nutritional Information:

Calories: 240

Fat: 4g

Carbohydrates: 38g

Fiber: 5g

Protein: 15g

Apple Slices with Almond Butter and Cinnamon

Ingredients:

1 medium apple, cored and sliced

2 tablespoons almond butter

1/4 teaspoon ground cinnamon

Instructions:

Arrange the apple slices on a plate or platter.

In a small bowl, mix the almond butter and cinnamon until well combined.

Dip the apple slices into the almond butter mixture and enjoy!

Nutritional Information (per serving):

Calories: 214

Fat: 14g

Carbohydrates: 20g

Fiber: 5g

Protein: 5g

Greek Yogurt with Berries and Honey

Ingredients:

1/2 cup plain Greek yogurt

1/2 cup mixed berries (such as strawberries, blueberries, and raspberries)

1 tablespoon honey

Instructions:

In a small bowl, mix the Greek yogurt and mixed berries until well combined.

Drizzle with honey and enjoy!

Nutritional Information (per serving):

Calories: 128 / Fat: 0g / Carbohydrates: 21g

Fiber: 2g / Protein: 11g

Shopping List:

Apples

Peanut butter

Greek yogurt

Honey

Cinnamon

Whole-grain bread

Avocado

Tomatoes

Cilantro

Lime

Salt

Whole-grain tortilla chips

Canned black beans

Salsa

Red onion

Garlic powder

Paprika

Cayenne pepper

Unsweetened cocoa powder

Dates

Almonds

Vanilla extract

Salt

Note: Please adjust the quantity of the ingredients according to your needs and preferences.

Protein:

Boneless, skinless chicken breast

Ground turkey

Wild-caught salmon fillets

Vegetables:

Broccoli florets

Carrots

Celery

Zucchini

Mushrooms

Red bell pepper

Garlic

Ginger

Onion

Baby spinach

Avocado

Cherry tomatoes

Cucumber

Red onion

Fresh parsley

Fruits:

Fresh berries (e.g., strawberries, raspberries, blueberries)

Pantry Staples:

Olive oil

Coconut oil

Apple cider vinegar

Balsamic vinegar

Dijon mustard

Low-sodium soy sauce

Honey

Garlic powder

Onion powder

Paprika

Cayenne pepper

Sea salt

Black pepper

Almond flour

Coconut flour

Unsweetened shredded coconut

Chopped nuts (e.g., almonds, pecans)

Dairy:

Feta cheese

Parmesan cheese

Eggs:

Large eggs

Miscellaneous:

Zucchini noodles

Chicken broth

Ground flaxseed

Unsalted butter

Stevia or monk fruit sweetener

Protein powder (e.g., whey protein, pea protein, hemp protein)

Please note that this list may vary depending on your personal preferences and dietary restrictions. It's always a good idea to check your pantry and fridge before going grocery shopping to avoid buying unnecessary items.

I hope this helps with your meal planning and shopping!

CHAPTER FOUR

STAYING ON TRACK

Mindset and Motivation

Motivation and a positive outlook are vital components of sticking to any diet or lifestyle change, including the Atkins diet. Keeping a positive attitude and staying motivated will help you stick to your objectives and make the necessary modifications to your eating habits.

Here are some suggestions for keeping motivated and having a positive attitude while on the Atkins diet:

Create attainable objectives: When beginning the Atkins diet, create attainable goals for yourself. Setting unrealistic goals might result in disappointment and dissatisfaction. Set smaller, more attainable goals to help you stay motivated and on track.

Maintain a good attitude and concentrate on the benefits of the Atkins diet. Remind yourself of the good things you're doing for your health and well-being.

Maintain a food journal: Maintaining a food diary can assist you in staying on track and holding yourself accountable for your food choices. It can also assist you in identifying any trends or triggers that are impeding your progress.

Make a plan: When you don't have time or healthy options accessible, planning your meals and snacks ahead of time might help you avoid making harmful food choices.

Maintain contact: Seek help from family, friends, or a support group. Having people around you who understand and support your objectives might help you stay motivated and on track.

Celebrate your accomplishments: Reward yourself when you meet your goals. However, be sure that your rewards are in line with your health and fitness objectives.

You can effectively follow the Atkins diet and reach your health and wellness objectives by staying motivated and having a positive outlook.

Overcoming Obstacles

Overcoming problems might be challenging, but it is doable with the appropriate mentality and tactics. Here are some pointers for overcoming obstacles:

Maintain a good attitude: Maintaining a positive attitude will help you stay motivated and focused even when faced with problems. Concentrate on your accomplishments thus far and appreciate your minor victories.

Set attainable objectives: Divide your major objectives into smaller, more attainable ones. This might help you stay motivated and track your progress.

Create a strategy: Make a strategy for achieving your objectives, including specific activities and timeframes you will specify. A well-thought-out strategy may help you stay organized and focused.

Seek help: For assistance and encouragement, contact family, friends, or a support group. Speaking with someone who knows your situation may bring both comfort and drive.

Remember that setbacks and challenges are a natural part of the process. Learn from them and use them to help you develop and become better.

Self-care: It entails taking care of yourself physically and psychologically by getting adequate sleep, exercising, and eating nutritious foods. Make time for things that you like and that help you unwind.

Stay adaptable: Be ready to change your plans and methods as required. Being adaptable might help you overcome unanticipated challenges and stay on track to achieve your goals.

Seek help and accountability: It can be difficult to keep motivated and accountable while working alone on a project. Seeking aid from family, friends, or a support group can provide the motivation and accountability required to overcome obstacles.

Consider hiring a coach or working with a dietician to assist you in staying on track and overcoming hurdles. A coach or dietician can give targeted advice and assistance based on your unique needs and goals.

Maintain your flexibility and adaptability: It is critical to remember that failures and struggles are a typical part of any path toward a goal. The ability to adjust and remain flexible in the face of hurdles is critical to conquering them.

If you discover that a specific method or approach isn't working for you, be willing to try new things and experiment until you find what does. Remember that growth is not always linear, and it is OK to make and learn from errors.

Finally, recognizing your victories, no matter how minor, will help keep you encouraged and inspired to continue conquering obstacles. Take time to recognize and enjoy your victories and development, and utilize these good experiences to drive your continuous efforts to achieve your goals.

Including Exercise in the Atkins Diet

Exercise can help with weight reduction, general health, and energy levels on the Atkins Diet. Here are some pointers to help you include exercise into your Atkins diet plan:

Begin Slowly: If you're new to fitness or haven't exercised in a long time, begin slowly and gradually build your intensity and length over time. This will aid in the prevention of injury and burnout.

Choose Activities You Will Enjoy: Working out does not have to be a hassle. Choose enjoyable activities such as walking, cycling, swimming, or yoga. This increases the likelihood that you will stick to your fitness plan.

Find a Workout Partner: Having a workout partner may help with motivation, accountability, and support. Consider collaborating with a friend or family member or enrolling in a group exercise program.

Change It Up: Repeating the same exercise program might become monotonous. Try new things or alternate between different forms of exercise, such as aerobic and weight training.

Make it a habit: Incorporate exercise into your daily schedule and treat it like you would any other essential appointment. When it comes to developing a good workout habit, consistency is essential.

Fuel your exercises: Make sure your body is getting the nutrition it needs to sustain your exercises. This might involve having a small meal or snack before activity, remaining hydrated, and refilling your body with protein and carbohydrates afterward.

By including regular exercise into your Atkins Diet plan, you may improve your weight reduction and general health while establishing a healthy lifestyle that is sustainable.

Exercise is a vital part of living a healthy lifestyle, and it may help maximize the advantages of the Atkins diet. Regular physical exercise can improve cardiovascular health, muscle mass, and metabolism, all of which can aid in weight reduction and control.

There are several ways to incorporate exercise into the Atkins diet. For example, you may begin by committing to 30 minutes of moderate-intensity exercise on most days of the week. Brisk walking, cycling, swimming, or dancing are examples of such activities.

Lifting weights or utilizing resistance bands, for example, can also be an efficient technique to develop muscle and enhance metabolism. Even if you're not exercising, this can help you burn extra calories throughout the day.

It's also worth noting that exercise might have an influence on your carbohydrate requirements. If you exercise on a regular basis, you may need to change your carbohydrate intake to ensure that your body has enough energy to sustain your exercise.

Staying hydrated and fueling your body with the correct nutrients are also vital for getting the most out of your workout regimen. To refill your energy resources, drink lots of water before, during, and after exercise, and eat a balanced meal or snack that combines protein and carbs.

Overall, including exercise in your Atkins diet may be an excellent approach to improving your health and reaching your weight reduction objectives. Before beginning any new fitness regimen, consult with your doctor or a trained nutritionist, especially if you have any underlying health concerns.

Here's an illustration:

Assume an Atkins dieter wishes to include strength training in their exercise program. They may schedule two 30-minute strength training sessions each week, concentrating on exercises that target key muscular groups such as squats, lunges, push-ups, and rows. They might also include 30 minutes of vigorous walking or cycling three times per week as cardio activity.

They might strive to consume a modest, high-protein breakfast or snack before exercising, such as a protein shake or a handful of almonds, to ensure they have enough energy for their exercises. They might replenish after their activity with a bigger meal that has a combination of protein, healthy fats, and carbs from non-starchy veggies.

Individuals must listen to their bodies and make the necessary modifications. If they become exhausted or develop muscular pain, they should reduce their workouts or take a day off to enable their bodies to heal.

Habits of a Healthy Lifestyle

Healthy lifestyle behaviors that can contribute to a successful weight reduction journey and complement the Atkins Diet include:

Regular physical activity: Including regular physical activity in your daily routine is critical for general health and weight control. Each week, try to get at least 150 minutes of moderate-intensity activity or 75 minutes of vigorous-intensity exercise.

Staying hydrated: Is essential for healthy health and weight reduction. Drink eight 8-ounce glasses of water every day, or more if you are physically active or in a hot climate.

Sleep: Getting enough sleep is critical to maintaining a healthy weight and general well-being. Aim for at least 7–8 hours of sleep every night.

Stress management: Because high levels of stress can contribute to overeating and bad food choices, it is critical to identify healthy strategies to handle stress. Meditation, yoga, deep breathing exercises, and indulging in hobbies and activities that you like are all examples of this.

Mindful eating: Being aware of your eating patterns might assist you in making better food choices and avoiding overeating. Paying attention to your hunger and fullness cues, eating deliberately and appreciating your meal, and avoiding distractions like television or your phone while eating are all part of this.

Balanced meals: It is critical to ensure that your meals are balanced and include a range of nutrient-dense foods such as vegetables, fruits, lean meats, and healthy fats when following the Atkins Diet. This will help your body get the nutrition it needs to function properly.

Portion control: Consuming too many calories, even while eating nutritious meals, can contribute to weight gain. To properly portion out your meals and snacks, use measuring cups, food scales, or other equipment.

You can support your weight reduction objectives while also improving your overall health and well-being by implementing these healthy lifestyle behaviors into your daily routine.

CHAPTER FIVE

HEALTH BENEFITS OF THE ATKINS DIET FOR SENIORS

Weight loss and weight management

Weight reduction and weight management are important components of the Atkins Diet because they can help people attain and maintain their ideal weight while also improving their overall health. Here is some weight reduction and weight control advice for the Atkins Diet:

Set attainable weight reduction goals: Setting attainable weight loss goals might help you stay motivated and on track. Determine a healthy and realistic weight reduction target based on your present weight, body composition, and lifestyle with the help of a healthcare provider or a qualified dietitian.

Keep track of your progress: Keeping track of your weight reduction progress will help you determine what works and what doesn't. Consider using a food journal, an app, or other monitoring tools to keep track of your weight, body measurements, and food intake.

Make good food choices: The Atkins Diet promotes whole, healthful meals, including lean protein, healthy fats, and nonstarchy veggies. Concentrate on including these nutrients in your diet while avoiding processed meals, sugary drinks, and snacks.

Exercise on a daily basis: Including regular physical exercise in your routine will help you lose weight and improve your overall health. Most days of the week, aim for at least 30 minutes of moderate-intensity activity, such as brisk walking, cycling, or swimming.

Drink enough water: Drinking plenty of water might help you feel full and prevent overeating. Aim for at least 8 glasses of water each day, and consider drinking water before meals to aid with hunger management.

Get adequate sleep: Sleep is essential for weight reduction and weight control since a lack of sleep can cause hormonal imbalances that encourage weight growth. Aim for a minimum of 7-8 hours of sleep every night.

Manage stress: Chronic stress can cause weight gain and make weight reduction more difficult. Consider implementing stress-reduction strategies such as meditation, yoga, or deep breathing exercises into your daily routine.

Blood Sugar Control

Controlling blood sugar levels is essential in the treatment of illnesses such as diabetes, hypoglycemia, and metabolic syndrome. Keeping blood sugar levels constant is also important for overall health since variations can cause tiredness, mood changes, and food cravings.

Some healthy lifestyle choices that can help with blood sugar regulation are as follows:

Balanced Meals: Consuming a variety of carbs, protein, and healthy fats will help manage blood sugar levels. It's critical to eat nutrient-dense, fiber-rich meals that digest slowly and give you long-lasting energy. Whole grains, fruits and vegetables, lean protein, and healthy fats like nuts, seeds, and avocado are all examples.

Portion Control: Even eating nutritious meals in large quantities might induce blood sugar rises. To avoid this, eat smaller, more regular meals throughout the day rather than a few large ones.

Exercise on a regular basis: Can enhance insulin sensitivity, which can help with blood sugar control. It is critical to find an activity that you like and include it in your daily routine.

Stress Management: Stress can induce blood sugar to rise by releasing stress hormones such as cortisol. Stress management techniques such as meditation, deep breathing, and yoga can help maintain blood sugar levels.

Adequate Sleep: Sleep deprivation can interfere with blood sugar homeostasis and raise the risk of insulin resistance. To maintain optimal blood sugar regulation, aim for seven to eight hours of sleep every night.

Heart Health

The Atkins Diet is good for your heart since it encourages you to eat healthy fats like avocados, nuts, seeds, and fatty fish. These fats can help lower cholesterol levels, lowering the risk of heart disease.

Furthermore, the Atkins Diet promotes non-starchy vegetables, which are high in fiber, vitamins, and minerals that promote heart health. The diet also restricts the use of processed foods, which are frequently heavy in salt, bad fats, and added sugars, all of which contribute to heart disease.

Following a low-carb diet, such as the Atkins Diet, has been found to improve a variety of heart disease risk factors, including blood pressure, triglycerides, and HDL (good) cholesterol levels. However, the long-term consequences of the Atkins Diet on heart health are still being explored, and it may not be appropriate for everyone, particularly those with pre-existing cardiac issues.

Adapting the Atkins Diet for Medical Conditions

Individual health concerns can be accommodated by tailoring the Atkins diet. Those with high blood pressure or heart disease, for example, may need to restrict their salt consumption, which includes selecting low-sodium protein sources and avoiding processed meals. Diabetes patients may need to regularly monitor their carbohydrate consumption and change their medication dosage accordingly. Before making any substantial dietary changes while pregnant or lactating, women should contact their healthcare professional.

A low-FODMAP variation of the Atkins diet may be advised for those who have digestive difficulties, including irritable bowel syndrome (IBS). FODMAPs are carbohydrates that are poorly absorbed in the small intestine and can aggravate IBS symptoms. Wheat, onions, garlic, and some fruits are rich in FODMAPs. A low-FODMAP Atkins diet would entail avoiding or restricting certain items in favor of low-FODMAP alternatives.

Overall, when adapting the Atkins diet for a specific health problem, it's critical to consult with a healthcare physician or certified dietitian to verify that nutrient demands are satisfied and health goals are accomplished.

Individuals suffering from particular medical disorders, such as diabetes or high blood pressure, may need to tailor the Atkins Diet to their unique requirements. People with diabetes, for example, may need to regularly monitor their carbohydrate consumption and alter their prescription dosages when they move to a low-carbohydrate diet. To make any required changes to the Atkins Diet, it is critical to engage closely with a healthcare expert, such as a registered dietitian or doctor.

People with high blood pressure should eat foods high in potassium and low in sodium, such as leafy greens, tomatoes, and avocados. A low-carbohydrate diet may also help decrease blood pressure, but it's critical to periodically monitor blood pressure readings and modify prescription dosages as required.

A modified Atkins diet that incorporates heart-healthy fats like olive oil and almonds while limiting saturated and trans fats may assist those with a history of heart disease or high cholesterol. Working with a healthcare expert to monitor cholesterol levels and adapt the diet is critical.

Pregnant women and toddlers should also consult with a doctor to verify that they are getting their nutritional needs met while on the Atkins Diet. It is critical that kids consume enough calories, protein, and necessary minerals for growth and development.

Overall, while the Atkins Diet may be a useful tool for weight reduction and health management for many people, it is critical to tailor the diet to individual requirements and health circumstances. A healthcare provider and a qualified dietitian can assist in ensuring a safe and effective transition to the Atkins Diet.

CHAPTER FIVE

CONCLUSION

Key Principles and Strategies: Recap

To summarize, the Atkins Diet is a high-fat, low-carbohydrate diet that can result in weight loss and improved health outcomes such as blood sugar management and heart health. The following are some crucial ideas and tactics to remember when following the Atkins Diet:

Limiting carbohydrate consumption to a specific quantity per day depends on your specific needs and goals. Incorporate healthy fats into your diet, such as avocado, almonds, and olive oil, to enhance satiety and improve blood lipid profiles. To assist muscle health and regeneration, consume a range of protein sources such as eggs, fish, chicken, and meat. Include non-starchy veggies in your diet to receive fiber as well as critical vitamins and minerals. Individualizing the diet to meet individual health needs and preferences, such as introducing more plant-based alternatives or adjusting protein and fat consumption,

Regular physical activity can help with weight loss and general health. drinking water and other low-carbohydrate beverages to stay hydrated. If you're following the ketogenic diet, keep an eye on your blood sugar and ketone levels. Always consult a healthcare expert before beginning any new diet or fitness regimen, especially if you have pre-existing medical concerns.

Motivation to Get Started

Congratulations on investigating the Atkins Diet as the first step toward bettering your health and well-being. Making lifestyle changes might be difficult, but keep in mind that modest actions can lead to large outcomes.

Set attainable objectives for yourself if you're feeling overwhelmed. This might be as easy as changing a high-carb snack for a lower-carb alternative or incorporating a quick stroll after supper a few times each week. Celebrate your accomplishments, no matter how minor they may appear, and use them as inspiration to keep going.

Remember that the Atkins Diet is not a fast fix, but rather a lifestyle modification that can result in long-term health advantages. Setbacks and blunders should not discourage you; instead, refocus and get back on course.

Finding a support system, whether it's a friend or family member who is also on the Atkins Diet, an online support group, or a trained dietician who can give direction and accountability, may also be beneficial.

Above all, pay attention to your body and prioritize your health. The Atkins Diet is only one tool in a bigger health and wellness toolbox. Take the time to figure out what works best for you and your specific requirements, and don't be hesitant to make changes along the way.

Keep in mind that you've got this!

Final Thoughts and Success Strategies

As you begin on your road to a healthy living with the Atkins Diet, keep in mind that change does not happen quickly. It's a slow process that demands effort, focus, and patience.

Here are a few pointers to keep in mind to help you succeed:

Set attainable objectives: Don't expect to lose a lot of weight in a short period of time. Instead, strive for 1-2 pounds of healthy weight loss every week.

Keep track of your progress: Keep track of your weight, measurements, and food consumption. It will help you stay accountable and inspired as you observe your progress.

Plan your meals: Spend some time planning your meals and snacks for the coming week. It would be simpler to stick to your diet if you had healthy food readily available.

Find assistance: Having a support system may make or break your road to a better life. Find individuals who can encourage and motivate you, whether it's a friend, a family member, or a support group.

Maintain an active lifestyle by including regular physical exercise into your daily routine to help burn calories, develop muscle, and enhance overall health.

Keep in mind that the Atkins Diet is not a one-size-fits-all strategy. Customizing it to your unique requirements and preferences can assist you in reaching your health and weight reduction objectives. You can make the Atkins Diet work for you and attain a better, happier life with effort and commitment.

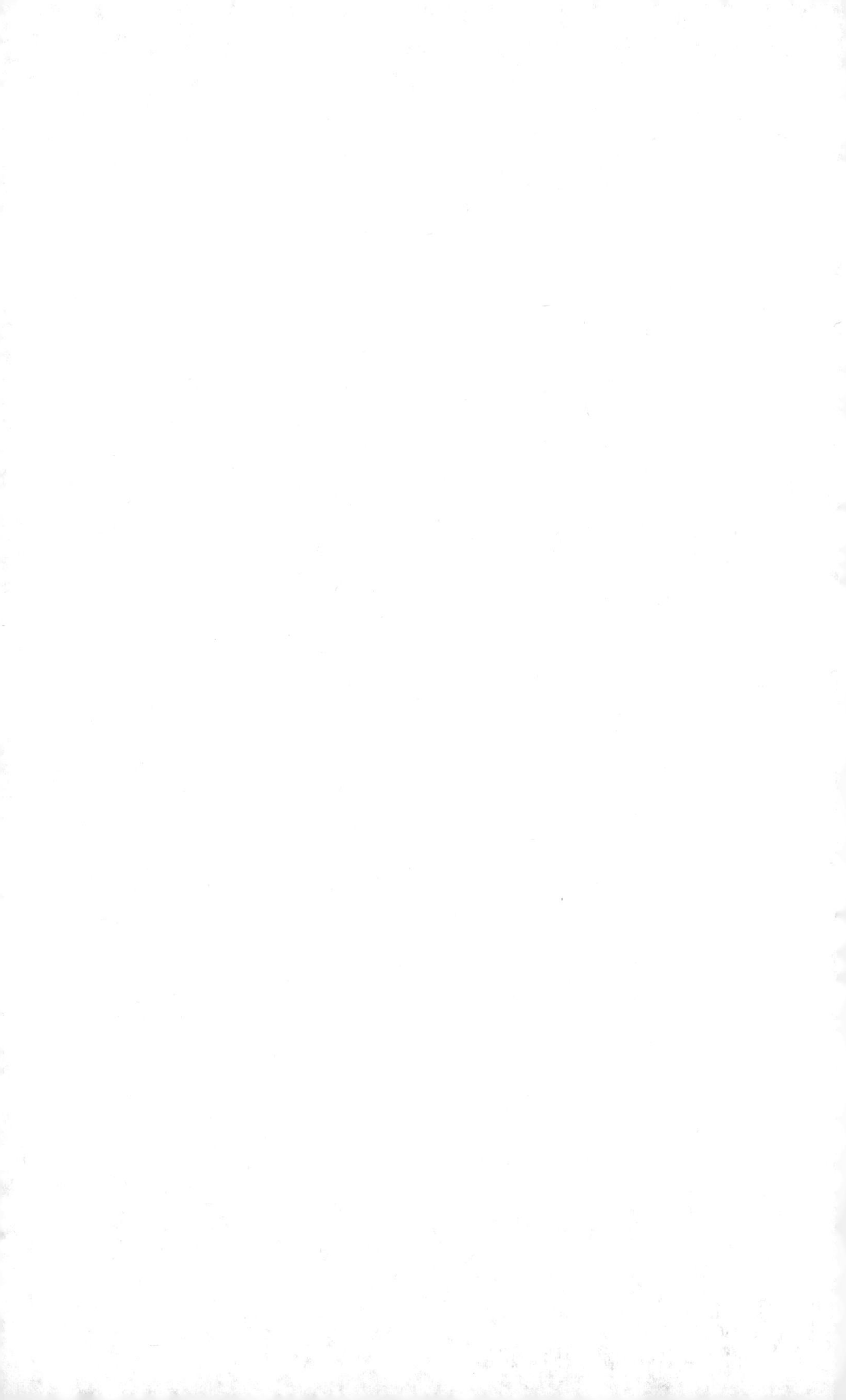

www.ingramcontent.com/pod-product-compliance
Lightning Source LLC
Chambersburg PA
CBHW061650250726
48659CB00004B/1444